FRUCTOSE INTOLERANCE DIET

A Beginner's 2-Week Step-by-Step Guide to Managing Fructose Intolerance, With Sample Fructose Free Recipes and a Meal Plan

Mary Golanna

mindplusfood

Disclaimer

By reading this disclaimer, you are accepting the terms of the disclaimer in full. If you disagree with this disclaimer, please do not read the guide.

All of the content within this guide is provided for informational and educational purposes only, and should not be accepted as independent medical or other professional advice. The author is not a doctor, physician, nurse, mental health provider, or registered nutritionist/dietician. Therefore, using and reading this guide does not establish any form of a physician-patient relationship.

Always consult with a physician or another qualified health provider with any issues or questions you might have regarding any sort of medical condition. Do not ever disregard any qualified professional medical advice or delay seeking that advice because of anything you have read in this guide. The information in this guide is not intended to be any sort of medical advice and should not be used in lieu of any medical advice by a licensed and qualified medical professional.

The information in this guide has been compiled from a variety of known sources. However, the author cannot attest to or guarantee the accuracy of each source and thus should not be held liable for any errors or omissions.

You acknowledge that the publisher of this guide will not be held liable for any loss or damage of any kind incurred as a result of this guide or the reliance on any information provided within this guide. You acknowledge and agree that you assume all risk and responsibility for any action you undertake in response to the information in this guide.

Using this guide does not guarantee any particular result (e.g., weight loss or a cure). By reading this guide, you acknowledge that there are no guarantees to any specific outcome or results you can expect.

All product names, diet plans, or names used in this guide are for identification purposes only and are the property of their respective owners. The use of these names does not imply endorsement. All other trademarks cited herein are the property of their respective owners.

Where applicable, this guide is not intended to be a substitute for the original work of this diet plan and is, at most, a supplement to the original work for this diet plan and never a direct substitute. This guide is a personal expression of the facts of that diet plan.

Where applicable, persons shown in the cover images are stock photography models and the publisher has obtained the rights to use the images through license agreements with third-party stock image companies.

CONTENTS

INTRODUCTION

Fructose intolerance is a condition where the body finds it difficult to digest fructose. According to studies, about 1 out of 20,000 to 30,000 individuals worldwide and annually are diagnosed with fructose intolerance.

Fructose is a type of sugar that naturally occurs in fruits, thus it's another term for fruit sugar. A more recent study also discovered that the human brain can also make fructose. This type of monosaccharide sugar is used to enhance flavors in food and drinks, this is why it's safe to assume that everyone has consumed fructose through meals.

When the body is unable to digest fructose, it leads to abdominal discomfort, bloating, and diarrhea. This, however, becomes almost unavoidable as most foods naturally have fructose. It should be noted that the thin line between fructose, glucose, and sugar should not be interchanged. Each plays an important role in the body; however, their uses and excesses should be understood by people to avoid underlying health issues.

If fructose is continuously ingested and not digested well, it may eventually damage the kidney and the liver. One remedy, however, is by eliminating as much fructose in your diet as possible. If you want to gain more knowledge regarding the concept of fructose intolerance and how to overcome it, continue reading. In this guide, you will learn about the following:

- The types of fructose intolerance
- The causes of fructose intolerance
- The symptoms of fructose intolerance
- How to overcome fructose intolerant
- Various diets to implement

THE NITTY-GRITTY OF FRUCTOSE AND FRUCTOSE INTOLERANCE

In case you have ever wondered if fructose intolerance has been around long enough, it should be understood that the term was coined in 1847 by Augustin-Pierre Duburnfait. The first case was identified and reported in 1956.

Fructose is the sweetest and most water-soluble of all sugars. This is a naturally occurring plant monosaccharide and provides four calories per gram. While fructose comes from fruits, it should be noted that the fructose from fruits is not enough to cause concern.

Having explained the above, it becomes quite confusing to understand how such a little calorie could lead to dangerous diseases. The individual tolerance for fructose differs universally, however, the standard American diet can be high enough to exceed the threshold for absorption even in those who do not have any compromise in their ability to absorb fructose. Free fructose has limited absorption in the small intestine, with up to one-half of the population unable to completely absorb a load of 25g. The average daily intake of fructose varies from 11 to 54 g around the world.

Hence, consuming fructose in large quantities leads to fructose intolerance. This occurs when cells on the outward surface of the intestine are unable to break down fructose efficiently. It is a digestive disorder in which absorption of fructose is impaired by deficient fructose carriers in the small intestine's enterocytes. This condition results in an increased concentration of fructose in the intestine.

Causes of Fructose Intolerance
Fructose Intolerance affects up to 1 in 3 people. This shows that this digestive order is gradually becoming widespread. From the aforementioned explanations, it is general knowledge that the large consumption of fructose would cause fructose intolerance.

Fructose is not only obtained from fruit; it is also produced commercially from corn or sucrose into a crystalline form which is used as an ingredient in packaged food and beverages. Apart from crystalline, it is in high fructose corn syrup (a mixture of the monosaccharide fructose and glucose). Crystalline fructose, high fructose corn syrup, and sucrose are termed "added sugar". They are added to food and beverages with the sole purpose of sweetness. Other reasons include: its properties could help improve texture, it blends well with beverages and it is good at absorbing water, etc. Hence, whenever you see the term "added sugar" as one of the nutrients, you can be perfectly assured that such a product contains a lot of fructose that shouldn't be consumed by anyone with fructose intolerance.

Fructose carriers found in erythrocytes are responsible for ensuring fructose is being directed to its necessary location. For anyone with a deficiency of carriers, fructose can build up in the large intestine leading to gut issues. Other causes include the imbalance of bad and good bacteria in the gut, excessive intake of refined and processed food, stress, inflammation, and pre-existing gut issues such as IBS (irritable bowel syndrome) amongst others, etc.

Symptoms of Fructose Intolerance
Symptoms are the body's mother tongue. Signs are in a foreign language- John Brown.

As a fructose-intolerant patient, numerous symptoms emanate from the body. These symptoms could help in analyzing fructose intolerance as the cause of discomfort. There are common and persistent symptoms according to research, such as nausea, bloating, gas, fatigue, and diarrhea. Other symptoms include cramping, abdominal pain, constipation, etc.

It should be noted that malabsorption of certain nutrients is also a symptom of fructose intolerance. When diarrhea is prolonged, the body expresses nutrient deficiency making the symptoms appear. Some of the nutrients affected are iron, calcium, and Vitamins C and E.
- Gas
- Cramping
- Intestinal Bloating
- Diarrhea
- Fatigue
- Headaches
- Brain Fog
- Constipation

When diarrhea occurs over prolonged periods, nutrient deficits and their symptoms may appear. The most common nutrients affected are folic acid, zinc, iron, calcium, vitamin c, vitamin e, and tryptophan.

Also, patients with fructose intolerance and malabsorption tend to show symptoms of mood changes and depression. A detailed study proves that fructose malabsorption is related to lower levels of "tryptophan." This plays a significant role in the development of depressive orders.

When you notice the above symptoms, be sure to contact a medical professional.

EVERYTHING YOU NEED TO KNOW ABOUT FRUCTOSE INTOLERANCE

While fructose intolerance gradually becomes widespread, research is carried out by medical institutions to help enlighten people. Numerous causes and risks have not been identified, however, according to 2011 research, it has been discovered that those between ages 1 and 5 years appear to have a higher intolerance to fructose than those between the ages of 6 to 10 years.

When this occurs in children (infants especially), they fail to grow and thrive at the expected rate. If undiagnosed and untreated in children, it becomes fatal. It is often diagnosed when babies start taking formula and baby food, as fructose could be used as a sweetener in this process.

Sometimes people do not have fructose intolerance but could develop it later in life. Anyone, irrespective of their age, could experience fructose intolerance.

A Cure We Never Knew We Needed

According to research, there is no cure or treatment that cures fructose intolerance. However, dietitians have made food plans that could help in reducing the risk and symptoms of fructose intolerance. If you want to get a diet that would help in overcoming and managing fructose intolerance, keep on reading!

Meanwhile, people are advised to avoid all fruits and numerous foods. They would need help and support to eat a balanced and healthy diet to avoid a lack of essential nutrients. Currently, fructose intolerance is permanent but it could be managed if the right precautions are taken by the individual.

Hence, the cure we all need is a well-studied and effective food plan which could help manage it. Also, a diet that makes food interesting for the individual.

Differences between hereditary fructose intolerance and fructose malabsorption

When speaking of fructose intolerance certain thin lines should not be blurred. They include Hereditary Fructose Intolerance and Fructose Malabsorption.

Hereditary Fructose Intolerance can be defined as a disorder in which a person lacks the necessary protein to break down fructose. This occurs when the body is missing an enzyme called Aldolase B. This is the substance needed to break down fructose. If a person with this digestive disorder eats fructose, it could lead to complicated chemical changes in the body. As a result, the body would be unable to change the stored form of sugar (glycogen) into glucose. This could lead to failure of the liver and a low level of sugar.

It is called hereditary fructose intolerance because it can be passed down through families. According to research, if both parents carry a nonworking copy of the Aldolase B gene, each of their children has a 25% (1 in 4) chance of being affected.

Hereditary Fructose Intolerance could be mild or severe

depending on the circumstance. People are advised to remove fructose and sucrose from their diet as it could help manage the condition. The severe form of hereditary fructose intolerance could lead to liver diseases and in such cases, the diet might not prevent severe liver disease in children. Some symptoms include vomiting, hyperventilation, liver or kidney failure, delayed growth, jaundice, etc. amongst many others.

On the other hand, hereditary Fructose Intolerance is more deadly than Fructose Malabsorption. Fructose malabsorption is otherwise known as dietary fructose intolerance. It is characterized by excessive gas and digestive discomfort.

The slight difference between hereditary fructose intolerance and malabsorption is that the cells of the intestine cannot absorb fructose normally. Besides, it cannot be passed through generations. Meanwhile, Hereditary Fructose Intolerance is caused by a deficiency of Aldolase B.

OVERCOMING FRUCTOSE INTOLERANCE

J ust like everything in life requires balance and moderation, so does fructose intolerance. Fructose intolerance is certainly a cause of concern but in-depth knowledge of the digestive disorder would help in managing the process.

Negative Effects of Fructose
Along with glucose, fructose is one of the two major components of added sugar. Some scientists and health practitioners are of the stance that fructose is the worst of the two, at least when consumed in excess.

While there are numerous benefits of fructose, there are a lot of negative effects when the level of fructose consumed is high. Many scientists believe that excess fructose consumption might be the key driver of many of the most serious diseases of today.

Fructose is metabolized differently by the body. While other cells in the body could make use of glucose, it is only the liver that could metabolize fructose in large amounts. Hence, when people consume it in large amounts, the liver tends to get overloaded, and afterward, the fructose turns into fat.

It should be noted that while it is common knowledge that excessive consumption of fructose causes a lot of diseases, research doesn't show the extent of the damage done. However, these are some of the effects of large fructose that could cause:

- Obesity and type II diabetes because it causes insulin resistance.
- High blood levels of uric acid lead to high blood pressure
- Accumulation of fat around internal organs increases the risk of heart diseases.
- Leptin resistance contributes to obesity.

Another thin line: It is clear that fructose has gotten fruit, however it should be emphasized that it is just a minor source of fructose compared to added sugar. The fruit has chewing resistance; which means that it takes a while to digest, hence the fructose hits the liver slowly. However, added sugar is extremely bad for people with fructose intolerance.

Baby Steps to Healthy Living
"You cannot control what goes on outside, but you CAN control what goes on inside"

Nothing is harder than having to cancel fruit smoothies and mouth-watering apples from one's diet. It's getting harder when hanging out with friends and I need to decline some mouth-watering dishes. Well, it's hard but extremely necessary for healthy living.

The first step to having control and managing fructose intolerance starts with the mind. As a fructose-intolerant patient, it is necessary to understand your body (the do's and don'ts). You need to understand:

- Peace of mind is extremely important than fleeting pleasures gotten from these dishes

- Food could also be made desirable even when you are on a diet.
- You are not missing anything from not eating these dishes.
- Stick to the food that is comfortable for your body system.

Having understood the aforementioned points, other points to take note of are the kinds of foods to eat and those to avoid. Always keep a food journal that would help you decide which fructose-containing foods bother you most. It should be known that some people can tolerate a small amount of fructose in their diets. Below is a table that could help with managing fructose intolerance:

Fruits
- It is preferable to eat fresh or frozen fruit to canned fruit.
- Tolerance depends on the person; the amount you eat at one time.
- Serving size is 1/2 cup—recommended 1 to 2 cups per day.

The following are recommended fruits to eat:

Intestine Friendly Fruits (Low Fructose)	Fruits To Avoid (High Fructose)	Questionable Fruit Juices/ Limit
Bananas, blueberries, strawberries, blackberries, coconut, kiwi	Apples, grapes, watermelon, dried fruits (mango, raisins)	Fruit juices or drinks, Apple cider, Apple juice
Avocado, oranges, lemons, raspberries, papaya	Plume, dates, pears,	Pear Juice, Applesauce, canned fruit in heavy syrup

N.B: All fruits contain fructose, however, there are some with harmful high fructose. Low-fructose fruits should be used as an alternative.

Vegetables
- Cooked vegetables are preferable as cooking causes loss of free sugars.

- The serving size is 1/2 cup, 1 cup; leafy green vegetable - recommended 1-1/2 to 3 cups per day.
- Tolerance depends on the person.

Intestine-Friendly	Foods to Avoid	Questionable Foods
Green beans, lettuce, cabbage, White potatoes, spinach	Asparagus, peas, tomatoes, onions, leeks, and shallot	
Sweet potatoes, carrots, Winter squash.	Okra, Mushroom, broccoli, Brussels sprout, garlic, tomato products (paste and ketchup)	

Other foods to avoid are wheat and any products made with it. This includes food such as pasta, couscous, or wheat bread. Rather make use of oats, rice, millet, or quinoa as a low-fructose alternative with the condition that they aren't sweetened with high-fructose corn syrup. Tofu and legumes are low in fructose but could cause intestinal gas.

Fructose Intolerant Patients could also eat all meat, fats, dairy, eggs, and sucrose (table sugar). However, when taking dairy products, caution is necessary to ensure that it isn't sweetened with high fructose corn syrup. Choosing soy milk, soy yogurt, rice milk, or almond milk is advisable. Anything with high fructose sweetness should be avoided.

Meanwhile, when buying products, always check ingredient lists carefully for high fructose sweetness. There are some labels to avoid. They include:
- Honey
- Agave syrup
- Invert sugar
- Maple-flavored syrup

- Sorghum
- Flavorings with sorbitol or fructose
- Desserts (ice cream, candy, cookies, bars) sweetened with fructose or sorbitol
- Cereal or other processed foods with sorbitol or fructose on the label.

N.B: Sorbitol is a sugar alcohol that is used as an artificial sweetener and is found naturally in fruits and fruit juices. It could be found in sugarless gum, sugar-free jelly/jam, and liquid medications. It normally creates similar symptoms as fructose-especially when they are ingested together.

Also, when eating out, it is extremely important to be cautious. Choosing the right restaurant is important, but when eating out, it is advisable to stick with salads and salad dressing. It's best to avoid soup and non-dairy products because they may be canned.

Having explained the different kinds of food to avoid and eat. Two kinds of diet could help in managing tolerance. They include Free Fructose and Low Fructose diets.

A low Fructose Diet is a diet that reduces the amount of fructose consumed by limiting or avoiding foods with excess fructose. Above is a table of low-fructose foods and vegetables. For 2-6 weeks, it is advisable to avoid high fructose food. During these weeks, signs of improvement would occur. Once signs improve, high fructose food could be slowly introduced to the diet in small amounts to determine personal tolerance. This is the reason for having a food journal/diary.

Free Fructose is a diet that completely expels the intake of fructose consumed by individuals. This diet is strictly advisable for people with hereditary fructose intolerance. This would help in managing intolerance.

THE DIET WE ALL NEED

Whether you have hereditary or dietary fructose intolerance, you may be able to do something to help your body deal with it and avoid the symptoms by following a diet that is specifically curated for your condition.

Before embarking on this diet program, it is best to consult first with your doctor and a nutritionist, so they can help you curate more tailored meal plans for you. One of the best ways to kickstart a diet program is by planning ahead of time. Doing this with your doctor and/or dietitian may help you plan better, especially with shopping for ingredients and following recipes to prepare your meals.

Here are steps you can follow during this two-week fructose intolerance program:

Week 1

• Prepare a food diary or journal
Use the information you'll get from your consultation with your doctor or dietitian in creating important notes and guides in your food diary or journal. Plot your daily meal plans and recipes here. Create a table where you can also include information about what you felt after each meal if you experience any discomfort or relief.

• Clean out your pantry

Another to motivate you as you start this journey is by cleaning out your pantry and removing all food items and ingredients that you will not be needing and may be substituted with better options, especially for your diet.

• Carefully list down your grocery list based on your meal plans

Create a grocery list by strictly adhering to your meal plans and goals. This way, you'll be able to plan well not only the things you have to buy but also your actual visit to the grocery.

Maximize the available tools you can use to buy your grocery needs. There are online tools like the Anylist app that you can use to create your grocery list with the help of those who either have the same condition as you or are also following a strict diet as you do.

It's also advisable that you group the ingredients and food items as how they are organized in your local grocery stores if you possibly can. This will be extremely helpful for you during your grocery run.

• Be mindful when doing your groceries

Now that you have properly listed out ingredients for your meals, it's time to plan out your grocery stroll. Not most people realize this, but even a typical grocery visit can actually become problematic for people who are strictly on a diet. Seeing all the food items you are supposed to avoid might tempt you to break from your diet and give in to the temptation of consuming them again.

To avoid this, make sure that you only visit the aisles or shelves where the ingredients you need are located. If you're familiar with the layout of your favorite grocery store, this will greatly help you avoid the aisles you need to avoid. If you're not familiar with the layout of the store, try to ask for assistance from the staff.

• Slowly transition your meals

It's always good if you can slowly transition to eating better by replacing one meal at a time until you are able to get used to consuming better options. For example, replace your snacks with healthier ones instead of the usual junk food.

Eventually, you may start replacing your main dishes with healthier options. This way, you can slowly transition into the diet and still enjoy it and avoid getting sick of it in your first few days.

In the first week, you should be able to consume the preferred meals for the entire week, continuing to the second week.

ACHIEVING YOUR GOALS

Week 2

- **Follow a stricter meal plan**

Now that you've somehow transitioned into the preferred diet meals, you'll need to be stricter in adhering to the program. The preparation you did the week before will help you to stay motivated to achieve your goals.

- **Find support from family and friends**

In case you feel the need to break away from your diet, try to seek support from family or friends, who can help you keep track of your progress and hold you accountable in case you are feeling tempted to break away from the program.

You may also want to try searching for a support group that has the same goals as you do, particularly sticking to a strict diet or those who also have fructose intolerance.

- **Take note of the changes in your body**

As your body gets used to the dietary changes you consume, you'll also experience changes in your body. Hopefully, most of them are good changes. Whatever they are though, make sure that you take note of them in your diary. This way, you'll be able to make a better assessment of how the diet program helped you during this

2-week period.

• Return to the doctor for an assessment

After the 2-week program, make sure that you make an appointment to visit your doctor to get an updated assessment. The notes you made in your food diary/journal will be a good basis for your doctor in assessing how the diet program has helped you.

SAMPLE RECIPES

Tahini Salmon

Instructions:
- 1/4 cup tahini
- 3 tbsp. fresh lemon juice
- 1 tsp. mashed garlic
- 1/4 tsp. salt
- 1/2 cup finely chopped cilantro
- 2 tbsp. roughly chopped toasted walnuts
- 2 tbsp. roughly chopped toasted almonds
- 1 tbsp. finely chopped onion
- 1 tsp. extra-virgin olive oil
- cayenne
- black pepper, freshly ground
- 1 lb. wild salmon skin removed, fresh or frozen

Instructions:
1. In a bowl, combine the tahini, 2 tbsp. of lemon juice, 3 tbsp. of water, mashed garlic, and 1/8 tsp. of salt; set aside
2. In a separate bowl, combine the cilantro, walnuts, almonds, onion, olive oil, cayenne, black pepper, and 1/8 tsp. of salt.
3. Fill the bottom of a steamer with water and bring it to a boil.
4. Season fish with 1 tbsp. of lemon juice.
5. Place it on a plate and put it on top of the steamer. Cover and cook, taking care to remove while the fish is still pink inside, about 3 to 4 minutes.
6. Remove the fish from the steamer, top with the tahini mixture, and then with the cilantro mixture.
7. Serve warm or at room temperature.

Salmon with Avocados and Brussels Sprout

Ingredients:
- 2 lbs. of salmon filet, divided into 4 pieces
- 1 tsp. ground cumin
- 1 tsp. onion powder
- 1 tsp. paprika powder
- 1/2 tsp. garlic powder
- 1 tsp. chili powder
- Himalayan sea salt
- black pepper, freshly grounded

Avocado sauce:
- 2 chopped avocados
- 1 lime, squeezed for the juice
- 1 tbsp. extra-virgin olive oil
- 1 tbsp. fresh minced cilantro
- 1 diced small red onion
- 1 minced garlic clove
- Himalayan sea salt to taste
- black pepper, freshly ground

Brussels sprout:
- 3 lbs. of Brussels Sprout
- 1/2 cup raw honey
- 1/2 cup balsamic vinegar
- 1/2 cup melted coconut oil
- 1 cup dried cranberries
- Himalayan sea salt
- black pepper, freshly grounded

Instructions:
To make the salmon and avocado sauce:
1. Combine cumin, onion, chili powder, garlic, and paprika seasoned with salt and pepper. Mix well before dry rubbing on the salmon.
2. Place the salmon in the fridge for 30 minutes.

3. Preheat the grill.

4. In a bowl, mash avocado until the texture becomes smooth. Pour in all the remaining ingredients and mix thoroughly.

5. Grill salmon for 5 minutes on each side or until cooked.

6. Drizzle avocado on cooked salmon.

To make the Brussel Sprout:

1. Preheat the oven to 375°F.

2. Mix Brussels Sprout with coconut oil. Season with salt and pepper.

3. Place vegetables on a baking sheet and roast for about 30 minutes.

4. In a separate pan, combine vinegar and honey.

5. Simmer in slow heat until it boils and thickens.

6. Drizzle them on top of the Brussels Sprouts.

7. Serve with the salmon.

Chicken Breast Delight

Ingredients:
- 1 tsp. dried oregano
- 1/2 tsp. rosemary
- 1/2 tsp. garlic powder
- 1/8 tsp. salt
- finely ground black pepper
- 4 chicken breasts

Instructions:
1. Remove any fat from the breasts.
2. Mix the remaining ingredients in a separate container.
3. Add the mixture to either side of the chicken.
4. Prepare a frying pan, lightly oil the pan, and set the stove to medium.
5. Add the chicken to the frying pan. Cook for 3 to 5 minutes on each face.
6. Cool the chicken for a couple of minutes after cooking.
7. Serve warm.

Steak with Olive Oil

Ingredients:
- 2 8-oz. grass-fed New York strip steaks, about 1-1/2-inch-thick, trimmed
- 3 tbsp. olive oil, divided
- 1 tsp. freshly ground black pepper, divided
- 1 tsp. kosher salt, divided
- 1 garlic clove, crushed
- 1 rosemary sprig
- optional: rosemary leaves

Instructions:
1. Place the grill pan over medium-high heat.
2. Brush a tablespoon of oil on the steak, then sprinkle with half a teaspoon of salt and another half teaspoon of pepper.
3. Put a tablespoon of oil into the pan, followed by a rosemary sprig and garlic.
4. Cook steak for about 9 minutes, or until preferred doneness is achieved. For every minute, turn the steak and baste it with oil.
5. Transfer the steak to a cutting board, letting it rest for 5 minutes.
6. Slice steak across the grain and place it on a platter. Drizzle with the juice from the cutting board and the leftover oil.
7. Sprinkle it with the remaining salt and pepper.
8. Upon serving, garnish with rosemary leaves if desired.

Mixed Vegetable Roast with Lemon Zest

Ingredients:
- 1-1/2 cups broccoli florets
- 1-1/2 cups cauliflower florets
- 3/4 cup red bell pepper, diced
- 3/4 cup zucchini, diced
- 2 thinly sliced cloves of garlic
- 2 tsp. lemon zest
- 1 tbsp. olive oil
- a pinch of salt
- 1 tsp. dried and crushed oregano

Instructions:
1. Preheat the oven to 425°F for 25 minutes.
2. Combine garlic and florets of broccoli and cauliflower in a baking pan.
3. Drizzle oil evenly over the vegetables. Season with salt and oregano.
4. Stir the vegetables to coat them evenly.
5. Place the pan inside the oven and roast for 10 minutes.
6. Add zucchini and bell pepper to the mix. Toss to combine.
7. Continue roasting for 10 to 15 minutes more until the vegetables turn light brown.
8. Drizzle lemon zest over vegetables and toss.
9. Serve and enjoy.

Spinach and Watercress Salad

Ingredients:
- 1 cup watercress, washed with stems removed
- 3 cups baby spinach, washed with stems removed
- 1 medium sliced avocado
- 1/4 cup avocado oil
- 1/8 cup lemon juice
- a pinch of salt

Instructions:
1. Pat dry the spinach and watercress. Remove the stem and separate the leaves.
2. On a large serving plate, combine the leaves of the watercress and the spinach.
3. Cut the avocado in half, then remove the pit. Peel the skin off from each side.
4. Slice the avocados into thin strips. Set aside.
5. Prepare the dressing by combining avocado oil and lemon juice.
6. Arrange the avocado strips on top of the watercress and spinach.
7. Season with salt and pepper.

Quinoa Lentil Salad

Ingredients:
- 2/3 cups dried brown lentils
- 2 cups water
- 1 cup quinoa
- 1 yellow sweet pepper, diced
- 1 shallot, chopped
- 1 bunch arugula, finely chopped
- 2 tsp. Dijon mustard
- 1/4 cup lemon juice
- 1/4 cup extra virgin olive oil
- 1/3 cup crumbled feta cheese
- 1 pinch salt
- 4 tbsp. fresh mint, chopped

Instructions:
1. Bring 2 cups of salt water to a boil in a saucepan.
2. Toss veggies into boiling salt water. Lower heat, and cook for 30 minutes.
3. Drain lentils and discard water. Set veggies aside.
4. Boil another batch of saltwater, and cook the quinoa in the pan.
5. In a bowl, mix pepper, salt, mustard, lemon juice, and oil.
6. Place veggies in a larger bowl, and pour the mixture.
7. Sprinkle mint and feta cheese over the salad.
8. Serve and enjoy

Baked Salmon with Dill and Lemon

Ingredients:
- 1-1/4 lb. salmon—king, sockeye, or coho salmon
- 1/4 tsp. black pepper, to taste
- 3 cloves garlic, minced or 1 tsp. garlic powder
- 1 tbsp. fresh chopped dill
- 2 tbsp. olive oil
- 1 tbsp. lemon juice

Instructions:
1. Preheat the oven to 350°F.
2. Grease a sheet pan with olive oil.
3. Season salmon on both sides with salt and pepper.
4. Combine olive oil, lemon juice, dill, and garlic in a small container.
5. In the baking dish, place the salmon skin-side down.
6. Drizzle the mixture over the fish and spread evenly on top.
7. Bake the salmon until the top is not opaque anymore, about 15-20 minutes.
8. To get a golden brown color on top, broil the fish at 425°F for a minute. Watch over it and check the middle temperature until it reaches 145°F.
9. Upon serving, garnish the salmon with dill and lemon slices.

Baked Salmon

Ingredients:
- 2 salmon fillets
- 6 cups of fresh spinach
- 2 tsp. coconut oil
- 1/4 tsp. garlic powder
- 1/4 tsp. turmeric
- 3 large cloves of garlic
- lemon juice
- salt
- pepper

Instructions:
1. Preheat the oven to 400°F.
2. Line a baking dish with parchment paper.
3. Marinate salmon fillets in lemon juice, coconut oil, garlic powder, turmeric, salt, and pepper.
4. Let it sit for a few minutes. This may also be done the night before to help the juices and flavor get into the salmon.
5. Once the oven is ready, bake salmon for 15 minutes.
6. Cook some of the garlic in a pan with coconut oil.
7. Add spinach and cook until ready. Season with salt and pepper to taste.
8. Take salmon out of the oven and put spinach beside it.
9. Serve and enjoy.

Crispy Chicken Thighs

Ingredients:
- 12 pcs. chicken thighs
- 4 tbsp. olive oil or avocado oil
- 2 tbsp. salt

Instructions:
1. Preheat the oven to 450°F.
2. Carefully rub the salt on the chicken thigh.
3. Place each thigh on a greased tray. Make sure there are spaces in between the thighs.
4. Drizzle the thighs with oil.
5. Bake in the oven until the skin is crispy, for about 40 minutes.
6. Serve and enjoy while hot.

Bacon Chicken Bites

Ingredients:
- 1 large chicken breast, large, cut into 22 to 27 small pieces
- 8-9 thin bacon slices, chop each into 3
- 3 tbsp. garlic powder

Instructions:
1. Preheat the oven to 400°F.
2. Use aluminum foil to line a baking tray.
3. In a bowl, place the garlic powder. Dip each chicken piece into the garlic powder.
4. Wrap a bacon piece around a chicken piece. After wrapping, arrange the bacon-chicken pieces on the baking tray.
5. Bake until the bacon becomes crispy, for about 25 to 30 minutes. About 15 minutes into baking, turn the chicken pieces.
6. Remove from the oven and arrange on a serving plate.
7. Serve and enjoy.

Thai Salad with Coconut Curry Sauce

Ingredients:
- 3 cups kale, chopped
- 2 cups napa cabbage, chopped
- 1 red bell pepper, chopped
- 1 cup carrots, shredded
- 1 cup mango, chopped
- 1/2 cup peanuts, chopped
- 1/2 cup cilantro, chopped

Dressing:
- 1 can low-fat coconut milk
- 1/4 cup creamy peanut butter
- 1 tbsp. yellow curry powder
- 1 clove garlic
- fresh lime juice
- 1-2 tsp. sriracha
- 1 tsp. kosher salt, or to taste

Instructions:
1. Place all the dressing ingredients in a blender. Blend on high speed until very smooth.
2. Place the dressing in a saucepan. Bring to a boil.
3. Allow simmering until reduced and thickened, for about 10 minutes.
4. Place the remaining ingredients into a large bowl.
5. Toss with the dressing and serve immediately.

Avocado and Quinoa Salad

Ingredients:
- 4 avocados cut into pieces
- 1 cup of quinoa
- 400 grams of chickpeas
- 30 grams of fresh parsley

Instructions:
1. In a pot, boil quinoa with 2 cups of water.
2. Reduce heat to a simmer, cover, and cook for 12 minutes until water is evaporated.
3. Fluff with a fork until grains are swollen and glassy.
4. Toss all the ingredients together.
5. Season with sea salt and black pepper.
6. Serve warm with lemon wedges and olive oil.

Roasted Veggies

Ingredients:
- 1/2 lb. turnips
- 1/2 lb. carrots
- 1/2 lb. parsnips
- 2 shallots, peeled
- 1/4 tsp. ground black pepper
- 1 tbsps. extra-virgin olive oil
- 6 cloves garlic
- 3/4 tsp. kosher salt
- 2 tbsp. fresh rosemary needles

Instructions:
1. First, cut vegetables into bite-sized pieces.
2. Set the oven to 400°F.
3. Mix all the ingredients in a baking dish.
4. Roast the vegetables for 25 minutes until brown and tender.
5. Toss and roast again for 20–25 minutes.
6. Serve and enjoy while hot.

Quinoa-Based Asian Salad

Ingredients:
- 2 cups uncooked quinoa
- 4 cups vegetable broth
- 1 cup edamame
- 1/4 cup green onion, chopped
- 1-1/2 tsp. fresh mint, chopped
- 1/2 cup carrot, chopped
- 1/8 tsp. pepper flakes
- 1/2 tsp. orange zest, grated
- 2 tbsp. fresh Thai basil, chopped
- juice from half an orange
- 1 tsp. sesame seeds
- 1 tsp. sesame oil
- 1 tbsp. olive oil
- 1/8 tsp. black pepper

Instructions:
1. Mix the broth and quinoa in a pan.
2. Set the stove to high. Place the pan.
3. Let the mixture heat up for 12 to 14 minutes.
4. After heating, cover the pan and wait for 4 minutes.
5. Place the mixture in a separate container. Add in the rest of the ingredients.
6. Let it cool down before serving.

CONCLUSION

Thank you again for getting this guide.

If you found this guide helpful, please take the time to share your thoughts and post a review. It would be greatly appreciated!

Thank you and good luck!

REFERENCES

20 foods high in fructose(That aren't only fruits and veggies). (n.d.). LIVESTRONG.COM. Retrieved September 15, 2022, from https://www.livestrong.com/article/30454-list-foods-high-fructose/.

Brown, J. (n.d.). The human brain makes fructose, researchers discover – here's why that might be a big deal. The Conversation. Retrieved September 15, 2022, from http://theconversation.com/the-human-brain-makes-fructose-researchers-discover-heres-why-that-might-be-a-big-deal-73258.

Burkhart, A. (2020, April 25). What is fructose malabsorption? Is it the same as fructose intolerance? Amy Burkhart, MD, RD. https://theceliacmd.com/what-is-fructose-malabsorption-is-it-the-same-as-fructose-intolerance/

Fructose (C6h12o6)—Structure, properties & uses of fructose. (n.d.). BYJUS. Retrieved September 15, 2022, from https://byjus.com/chemistry/fructose/.

Fructose-free diet. (n.d.). GI for Kids. Retrieved September 15, 2022, from https://www.giforkids.com/fructose-free-diet/.

Fructose intolerance: Symptoms and management. (2022, March 11). https://www.medicalnewstoday.com/articles/fructose-intolerance.

Fructose malabsorption: Symptoms, management, and more. (2017, September 19). Healthline. https://www.healthline.com/health/fructose-malabsorption.

Hereditary fructose intolerance: MedlinePlus Genetics. (n.d.). Retrieved September 15, 2022, from https://medlineplus.gov/genetics/condition/hereditary-fructose-intolerance/.

Larry. J (2021, September 6). Blood Type Diet: A Beginner's Overview and 3-Week Step-by-Step Guide with Sample Curated Recipes, Blood Types Explained.

What is fructose intolerance? (2021, March 1). Cleveland Clinic. https://health.clevelandclinic.org/what-is-fructose-intolerance/.

Made in the USA
Las Vegas, NV
27 December 2024

15468620R00026